**Question:**
*How difficult is it to find the Press Points for backache, headache, sinus trouble, etc?*
**Answer:**
You will be amazed how fast you will locate them in your own or somebody else's feet. Just read the easy-to-follow instructions and look at the pictures.

**Question:**
*Can it be harmful?*
**Answer:**
No. It is beneficial to children as well as adults.

**Fact:**
As you start feeling the soothing benefits, Press Point Therapy grows on you. The results speak for themselves.

**Remember:**
People, when cranky, love the treat to the feet!

*Sandra M. Dolber*
California State Certified
Massage Therapist

# PRESS POINT THERAPY

## G. BENDIX

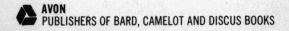

AVON
PUBLISHERS OF BARD, CAMELOT AND DISCUS BOOKS

AVON BOOKS
A division of
The Hearst Corporation
959 Eighth Avenue
New York, New York 10019

First Avon Printing, August, 1978

AVON TRADEMARK REG. U.S. PAT. OFF. AND IN
OTHER COUNTRIES, MARCA REGISTRADA,
HECHO EN U.S.A.

Printed in the U.S.A.

**DEDICATED**

to the men and women who,
during the last 5,000 years,
have searched for and discovered
the knowledge that helps us today.

# CONTENTS

## PART III

## THE SIX HEALTH ROUTINES

## PART IV

## HOW TO TREAT THE DIFFERENT AREAS OF THE BODY                                85

# FOREWORD

Press Point Therapy helps; it has helped those in the know for generations. Dedicate a few extra minutes a day to your health. There is no better investment.

> Young or old,
> Better than gold
> The greatest wealth
> Is your good health.

Clean air, vitamins and rest are as important as are regular checkups. There is no one answer or remedy for all that ails us. A bad tooth might cause pain anywhere in the body. Many headaches can be traced to the eyes. Emotional upsets may result in disrupting the digestive system or some other important body function.

# PART I

## WHAT TO LOOK OUT FOR AND WHY

### HOW DOES PPT HELP?

Nerve-like connecting pathways to all parts of the body are closest to the surface and easiest to locate in the feet. The connector points to glands, nerves and organs are called press points.

Various grips permit us to reach and treat tender spots in the feet. That relaxes and normalizes functions, and stimulates circulation.

How and where to do this is described carefully in this book and shown in pictures. Acquaint yourself with the different routines, learn the grips, and follow all the instructions closely. The results will speak for themselves.

## YOUR BODY'S ALARM SYSTEM –
## MAKE IT WORK FOR YOU

The body's warning signals are pain, nausea, dizziness, etc. When these symptoms appear, it is already quite late because many conditions of poor health take some time to develop.

## PPT'S AIM IS TO ANTICIPATE THESE
## WARNING SIGNALS

PPT will help discover many potential physical complications in their early stages or almost before they occur. Awareness of a condition in time often facilitates fast improvement. Treat according to the directions you find in this book. You will be amazed at how many conditions Press Point Therapy will take care of.

In case of serious or persistent symptoms, consult your doctor. Our great enemy, cancer, sends out only faint warnings. Know them. Get a bulletin from the American Cancer Society.

# CAN WE DIAGNOSE?

I would like to make it clear that regardless of how proficient those using PPT may become, and how much they may help themselves and those around them, all they are doing is helping people to relax, enabling conditions to normalize. It is done by stimulating the press points of glands, nerves, organs, etc.

Please do not try to act like a doctor. There is only one way to become an M.D.: one must spend many long years studying, learning, practicing.

Just do your routines and you will be richly rewarded by the knowledge that you are helping. The satisfaction you derive, and the acclaim of your friends and relatives are all one should expect.

# THE EXACT LOCATION OF GLANDS AND ORGANS

There is no exact location for anything in our body. Approximate location is a better description. You must consider that certain glands and organs are virtually on top of each other.

For that reason, it is wise to refer to areas as stomach area or bladder area. Once we discover one or several tender points, we treat the area. That generally will take care of the pain.

# IMPORTANT WARNING TO BEGINNERS

Glands, nerves and organs not used to this kind of stimulation need 8 to 15 days break-in time. When you treat any part of the body, especially if it is not working well, you cannot bully it into good behavior.

At first, you treat it very gently; next give it a two day rest; then work it gently again. That is the only way you will find relief or eventual cure. You still may get some kind of reaction during the first few treatments.

This has to do with the constitution of a person; active people need less break-in time. Beginners should start with the Break-In Routine.

# THE SIX HEALTH ROUTINES

## THE CHECK-OUT ROUTINE

Employ this once a week to discover possible trouble spots, regardless of how well you feel. Mark one day each week for this purpose on your calendar. You will be able to discover many possible health complications in their early stage, or almost before they occur.

Awareness of a possible condition in time often facilitates fast improvement. Always have a paper and pencil handy to take notes about the locations of tender spots you discover, or memorize them. Another feature of this once-a-week Check-Out Routine is the stimulation of points not covered by other routines. It will take 15 to 20 minutes for each foot at the beginning. Once you have practiced it a while, less than 10 minutes will be required. See page 47.

## THE MAINTENANCE ROUTINE

Employ this every second day for good circulation and to keep glands, nerves and organs stimulated. This regular practice relaxes and normalizes functions, stimulates circulation. It will take 8 to 10 minutes for each foot at the beginning. After a few weeks it will take only 3 to 4 minutes. See page 67.

## THE PICK-UP ROUTINE

Try this 3-4 minute routine for that tired, worn-out feeling. See page 73.

## THE CONDITION TREATMENT ROUTINE

This routine is employed for an upcoming or existing condition of poor health. Once a tender point is discovered, try to identify its source in the body by using the big map. Work on the area of the foot according to instructions. If you cannot identify the reason, just treat it according to area instructions. If that does not help soon, see your doctor. See page 77.

## THE MATURE PEOPLE ROUTINE

Its purpose is to delay the signs and effects of aging and improve existing conditions. See page 84.

## THE RELAXATION ROUTINE

This is to alleviate nervous tension and mental and emotional stress. See page 84.

## BREAK-IN ROUTINE –
## FOR NEWCOMERS TO PRESS POINT THERAPY

Cut your fingernails short; see picture No. 10. This is not necessary if you work with the instrument only. You cannot be gentle enough the first time you give yourself, or someone else, a foot treatment.

Follow the Check-Out Routine. Press firmly enough, but once only, for the pressure to be felt. Be very careful not to produce pain from the pressing itself. Press Point Therapy is effective when done with the sincere desire to help either yourself or someone else. This means no talking, smoking or even permitting your thoughts to wander during a Press Point Therapy session. You have to concentrate on what you are doing.

Allow plenty of time and press everywhere, making sure you reach every possible trouble spot, but once only. Make a note of where you found a tender point. Then wait two days, or at least one day in the case of an active person. You can now press the points two times and a bit more firmly.

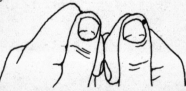

No. 10 Cut your fingernails, especially your thumbnails short.

Sex glands, kidneys, liver, and pancreas, see pictures Nos. 44 and 45, sometimes act up when receiving their first or their first few treatments. Once used to Press Point Therapy, these press points can be worked harder.

Right foot No. 45

Left foot

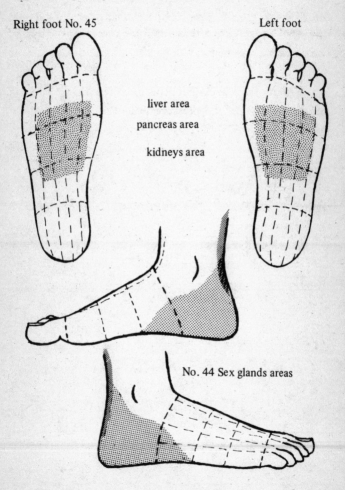

liver area

pancreas area

kidneys area

No. 44 Sex glands areas

Areas for the sinuses, hayfever, headaches, hemorrhoids and spine, see pictures Nos. 46, 47 and 49, actually can be treated a little more firmly right away.

Elderly and delicate persons should consider the first two weeks as break-in time. Active persons will adjust to Press Point Therapy in about a week.

No. 46 Spinal area

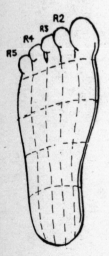

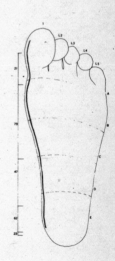

Cervical vertebrae

Thoracic vertebrae

Lumbar vertebrae

Sacrum

Coccyx

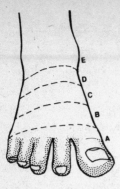

No. 47 Sinus, hayfever and headaches, in Section A

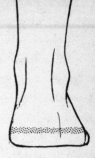

No. 49 Bony edge in back of feet; hemorrhoid area.

## THE IMPORTANCE OF THE CHECK-OUT ROUTINE

Searching for tender spots and finding them is half the battle. These connecting points, often as small as the point of a needle, have to be checked once a week. There is no telling where you will discover a sore spot. If you can remember, fine. Otherwise, write it down. Once past the break-in period, give the tender area a daily workout. Please do not be too gentle with yourself. The workout of a tender spot has to hurt. On the other hand, do not overdo it to the point where the pain becomes unbearable.

# THE CHOICE: INSTRUMENT OR THUMB PRESSURE

Beginners will find it easy to work with the simple instruments. See pictures Nos. 6 and 7. It does not require any special skill. Just follow the instructions, look at the pictures and you will find it easy.

Please have patience searching for tender or painful points. The most important part is finding the spots where our body is crying for help. Pay close attention to locating existing or future trouble spots. Next, treat them according to instructions.

## TO HELP OTHERS

Professional therapists work with their hands, mainly the thumbs. You have enough strength in your fingers, so by all means learn how to work with them. Read the easy-to-follow, explicit instructions in this book. When searching or working around the toe or pad area, employ the instrument.

## WHY THERE IS A VARIETY OF GRIPS

So that you may experiment and find the one best suited for you.

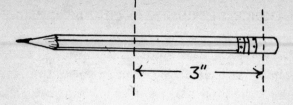

No. 7 Cut a pencil to about 3". Cut off 2/3 of the eraser or it will break when pressed down and moved in a circle.

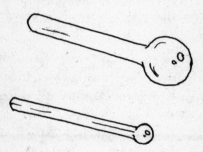

No. 6 Shorten a plastic cocktail stirrer to about 3"

## TOO LITTLE OR TOO MUCH STRENGTH

Be warned — do not bruise yourself or others. To find
tender points is a question of technique; strength alone will
not do it. When treating someone else, watch his or her face
for any reaction. The person should never wince from pain
while you are searching. Just make sure you reach every
possible spot to locate tender points.


## YOU DISCOVER A TENDER SPOT

Once you find the tender or sore press points that are
crying for help, memorize them. Look at the big map and
try to identify the pain, or at least the area where it origin-
ates. Read up in the book how to treat that area. The only
way to help is by pressing and rubbing and that often hurts.
There is nothing you can do about that. Put up with it
knowing that it will help. Often relief comes fast.


## HOW LONG WILL IT TAKE

A condition existing for an extended period of time
probably will take longer to improve.

# PART II

## THE TECHNIQUE MADE SIMPLE AND EASY TO LEARN

### HOW TO SIT

The three sitting positions for do-it-yourselfers are: On a chair, on the floor, or on the side of a bed. See pictures Nos. 1 to 4. In the beginning, your leg will get tired in an unaccustomed position. Just switch feet as necessary.

Some persons lean forward when treating their own feet, others lean back. Everybody has to develop his or her. own position. Try a few, and you will find one comfortable for you.

To treat others see picture No. 5.

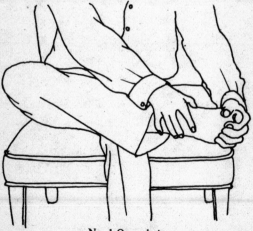

No. 1 On a chair

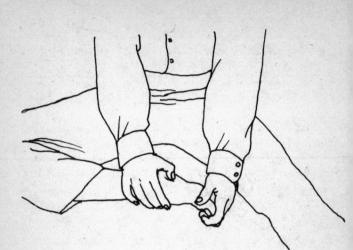

No. 2 On the floor

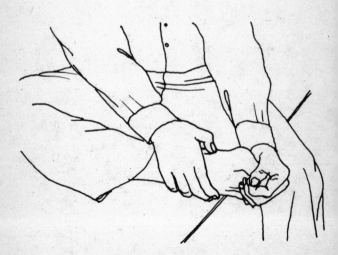

No. 3 On bed right foot

26

No. 4 On bed left foot

No. 5 A good way to hold when helping others

# THE DIFFERENT GRIPS

## THE MAIN GRIP

For the main grip, use only the side of thumb, next to the quick, not the fleshy part. See picture No. 10. Bend thumb and press down in a hooking-like motion. See pictures No. 11 and No. 12. Keep thumb locked in this position exerting pressure downwards, then move locked thumb in a circular motion. Next, advance one quarter of an inch and repeat. This is the most important of all grips. Practice it.

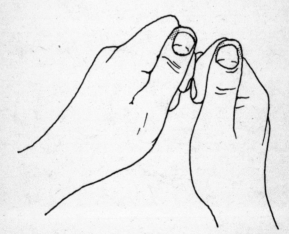

No. 10 Keep nails short. Employ shaded area for pressing.

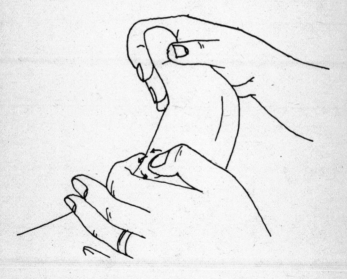

No. 11 Do-it-yourselfers

No. 12 Helping someone else

## THE MAIN GRIP WITH INSTRUMENT

Do-it-yourselfers and newcomers to Press Point Therapy feel more comfortable employing an instrument for it requires less know-how. See pictures No. 13, No. 7, No. 8 and No. 9. Press down and use a circular motion. Next, advance ¼" and repeat.

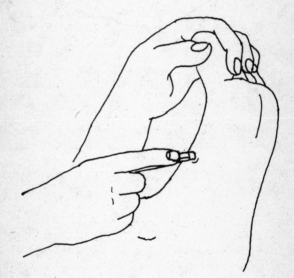

No. 13 Hold the instrument short

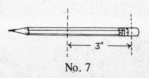

No. 7

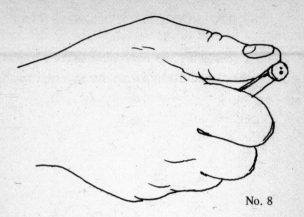

No. 8

Hold the instrument short for good leverage and so it won't break

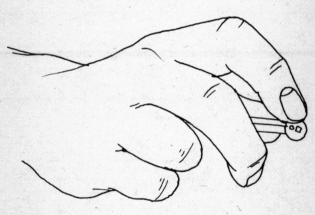

No. 9

# THE AUXILIARY GRIP WITH INSTRUMENT

The instrument is especially recommended for the toe section; it reaches better into every corner making sure the area has been checked thoroughly. See pictures No. 16, No. 17 and No. 18.

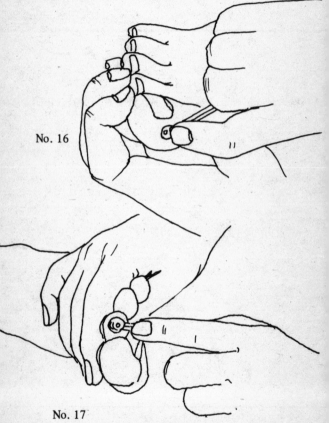

No. 16

No. 17

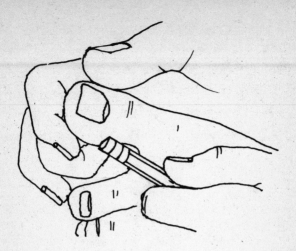

No. 18

## THE AUXILIARY GRIP

This is the auxiliary grip to the main grip. When you work around the toes, you find spots and corners hard to reach, where the toes are connected to the foot and also the sides of the toes. See pictures No. 14 and No. 15, on next page. Employ what is most convenient for you, the index or the middle finger. Use a twisting, screwing, or turning motion, making sure you cover every spot in the area. Advance less than ¼" at a time, especially around the big toes and between toes.

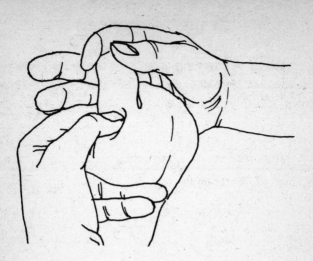

No. 14

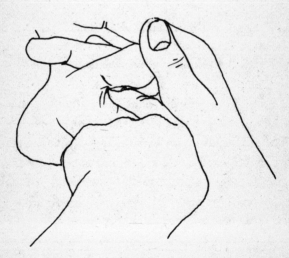

No. 15

# THE THREE FINGER GRIP

The three finger grip is used on the "ledge" between the toes and the ball of the foot. See picture No. 19. Press down, lock grip, and use circular motion. Cover full width from big toe to small toe. Use the same grip gently on top of the foot, but lengthwise between tendons. See picture No. 20. If using instrument apply strongly on the bottom of the foot, gently on the top.

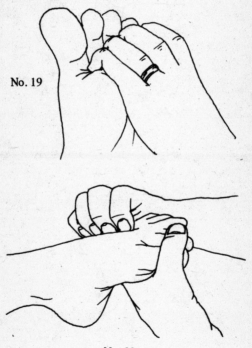

No. 19

No. 20

# THE KNUCKLE GRIP FOR THE MAINTENANCE
## ROUTINE ONLY

Employ either the knuckle of the thumb or the knuckles of the index and middle fingers. See pictures No. 21 and No. 22. It is used between the ball of the foot and the heel. Rub slowly up and down exerting pressure, touching every point at least twice. With instrument see picture No. 23.

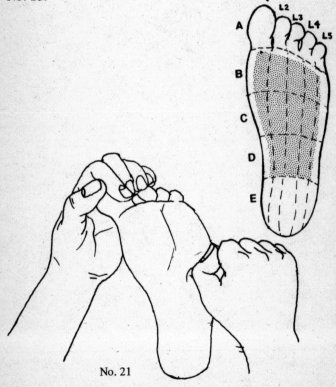

No. 21

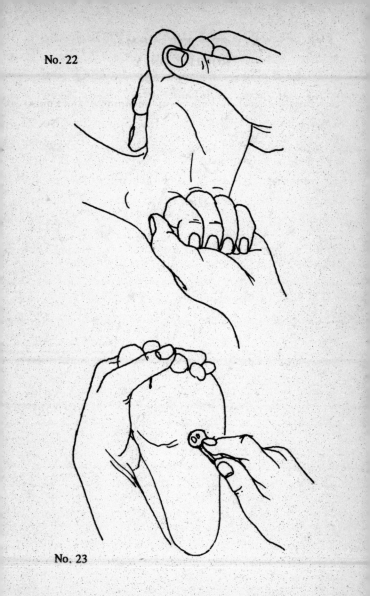

No. 22

No. 23

# FOR THE CHECK-OUT ROUTINE ON THE SOLE
# OF THE FOOT

Employ the main grip, never a *knuckle grip*. See picture No. 24. With instrument see picture No. 23, on previous page.

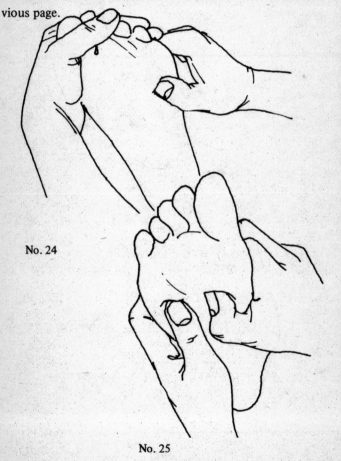

No. 24

No. 25

# HEEL KNOCK

There are three ways to reach the bony edge of the heel. Employ the main grip vigorously. Knock the foot against the floor, making sure you touch every spot. Or employ the instrument energetically. See picture No. 32.

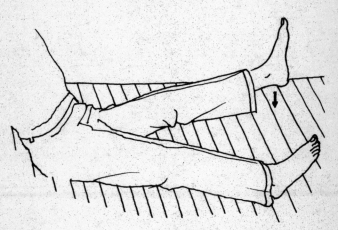

No. 32

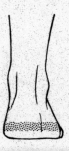

BACK

Indicates bony edge of heel.

## THE SIDE KNUCKLE GRIP

The side knuckle grip employs the side of the knuckle of the thumb or forefinger for the outside and inside of the heel. See pictures No. 30, No. 31 and No. 44. You can also use the main grip. See picture No. 29, or the instrument.

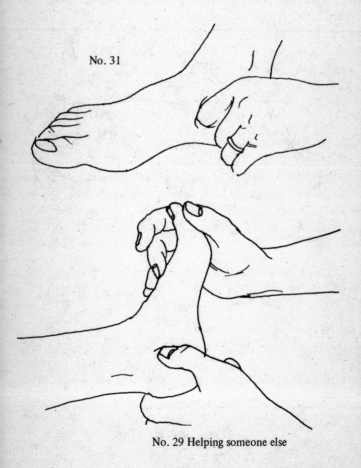

No. 31

No. 29 Helping someone else

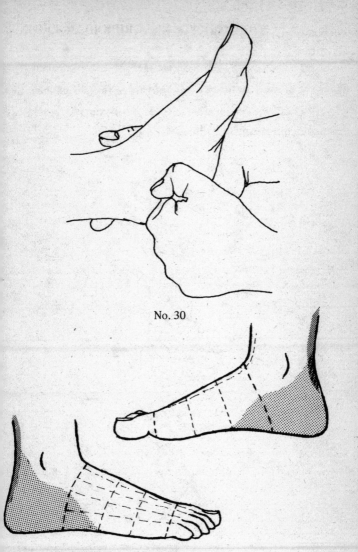

No. 30

No. 44

# THE THREE RELAXATION GRIPS

## THE FOOT TWIST

Loosen up by twisting foot three times each way. See pictures No. 35 and No. 36 for do-it-yourselfers, No. 37 for helping someone else.

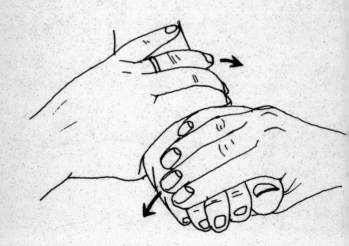

No. 37 Helping someone else

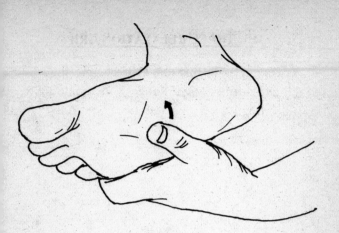

No. 35 Hook under

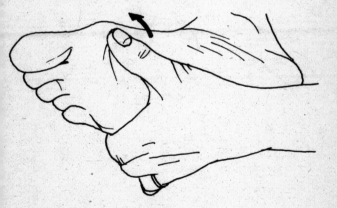

No. 36 Push with thumb

# THE HEAD RELAXATION GRIP

Take one of the big toes between your thumb, fore-finger, and middle finger. Rotate it in a wide full circle carefully right and left, till it feels loose. See picture No. 38

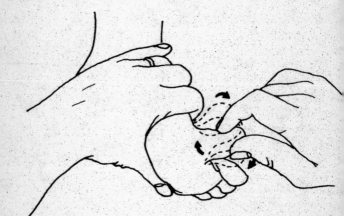

No. 38

# THE FULL RELAXATION GRIP

Put one hand above the two ankle bones, holding your leg. With the other hand, take a firm hold of your five toes, or hold the foot from below. See picture No. 39. Rotate your foot at the ankle in a wide circle, right and left, slowly and carefully, till the foot feels loose. Helping someone else, see picture No. 40. Always work both feet.

No. 39

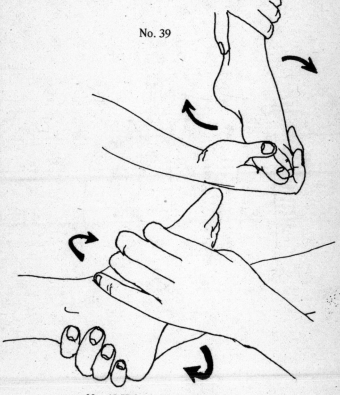

No. 40 Helping someone else

## WIND UP

After you have completed the three relaxation grips, inhale *deeply* through your nose, filling your lungs with fresh air, as much as possible. Exhale slowly but completely through your mouth. Repeat at least six times. See picture No. 41.

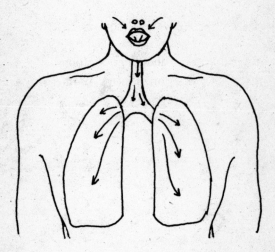

No. 41

# PART III

## THE SIX HEALTH ROUTINES

### THE CHECK-OUT ROUTINE

Employ once a week, regardless of how well you feel. Mark one day each week for this purpose on your calendar. You will be able to discover many possible health complications in their early stage, or almost before they occur.

Awareness of a possible condition in time often facilitates fast improvement. Always have a paper and pencil handy to take notes about the locations of tender spots you discover, or memorize them. Another feature of this once-a-week Check-Out Routine is the stimulation of points not covered by other routines.

If not indicated otherwise, work each area not less than two times, preferably three times, but not more than that.

If your leg gets tired in the unaccustomed position, just switch feet as necessary.

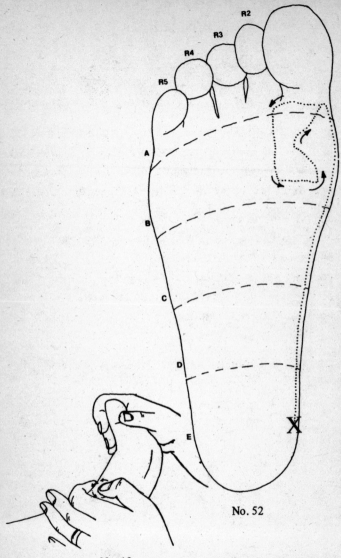

No. 52

No. 12

Rub feet vigorously. Start with your right foot at the X, as shown in picture No. 52. Use main grip with instrument or thumb, see pictures No. 11, No. 12 and No. 13. Progress no more than ¼" at a time. Follow the dotted line along the instep bone where the press points for the spine are located.

When you reach the big toe, follow the guide line along the groove where the big toe connects with the foot, to the end of the big toe. Use the instrument. As the dotted line shows, you follow the thyroid gland detour and end up, where you left off, at the big toe.

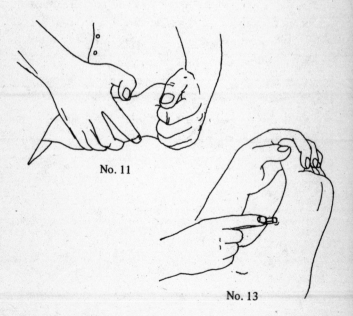

No. 11

No. 13

The press points for the head and the neck are located mainly in the big toes and in the remainder of section "A" right and left foot.

On the toes employ the auxiliary grip, preferably using the instrument, see pictures No. 14, No. 15, No. 16 and No. 17. Advance in small steps, less than ¼" at a time.

This is your weekly Check-Out Routine and you want to be sure you touched every possible spot twice, if not three times. Check every nook and corner between the toes. That is not easy, but everybody reaches the places eventually.

As you work along the press point line, as indicated, searching for tender spots and stimulating as you go, you will find beneath each big toe a press point to the pituitary gland. You will know at once when you touch it. The press points to the pituitary gland are always tender. That is normal, no reason to worry. Never forget to give three good pushes to this master gland even though it will hurt a little. Finish with the toes.

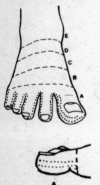

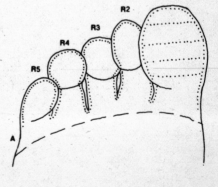

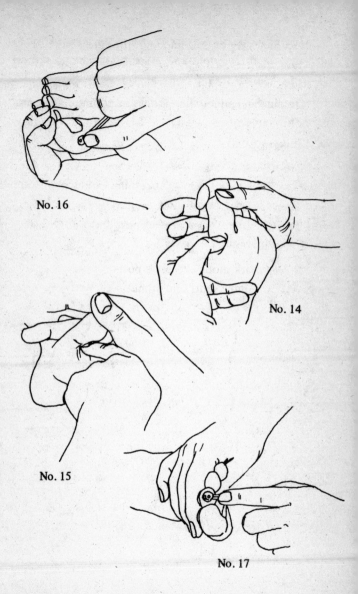

No. 16

No. 14

No. 15

No. 17

Proceed to the dotted line indicating the "ledge" between toes and ball of the foot. Use the three finger grip, see picture No. 19, or the instrument. Press firmly and according to the size of the foot from 4 to 8 times. Then on top of the foot use same grip, see picture No. 20, lengthwise and more gently.

Now rub, exerting pressure downward with a flat hand on top of the foot, while proceeding from toenails to ankle, covering the full width of the top of the foot. Release pressure, return to the starting point at the toes, repeat six times. See picture No. 50.

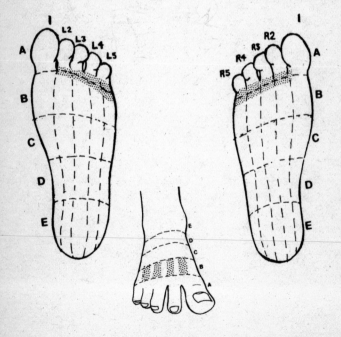

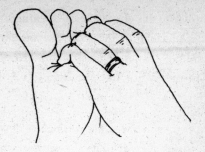

No. 19

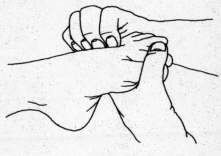

No. 20

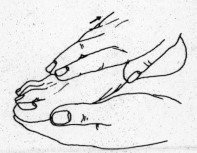

No. 50

Back to the bottom of the foot. Employ either the main grip, or the instrument, see pictures No. 23 and No. 24. Go from the ball of the foot to where the heel starts. *Never* use the knuckle grip for the Check-Out Routine on the sole. Look at the dotted lines and keep about 1/3" distance between the lines. That sounds very simple, and so it is, but . . . you are now covering a wide area, containing the press points for numerous glands, organs, nerves, etc. See picture No. 53 page 56. You are also treating with a dual purpose. First, you are searching to find possible future trouble spots. Next, you are trying to stimulate the press points to all those internal parts, usually not stimulated any other way.

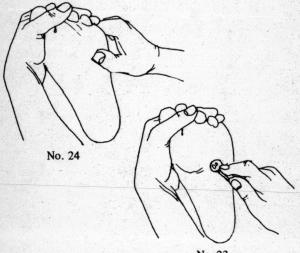

No. 24

No. 23

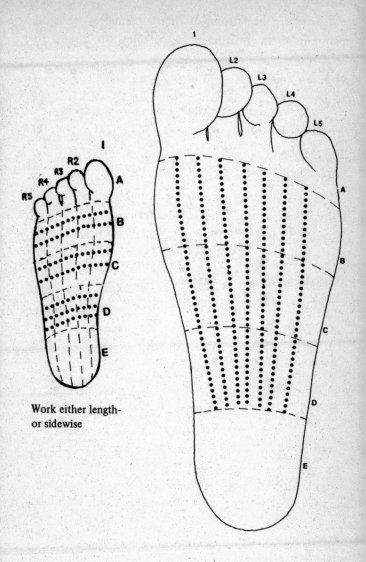

Work either length-
or sidewise

Please look at the body map; do you realize now how many press points are in the sole of each foot? Work this area with dedication and deliberation. Make sure you reach where you are supposed to.

When you use your thumb or the instrument for a Check-Out Routine to the sole of the foot, keep your forward motions to no more than 1/4" at a time, press firmly and keep about 1/3" distance between the lines.

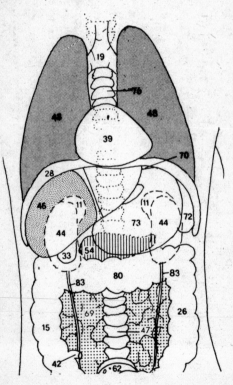

The dotted guide line now takes you to the bottom part of the heel (the pad) covered with thick skin. Use the instrument, see pictures No. 26 and No. 27.

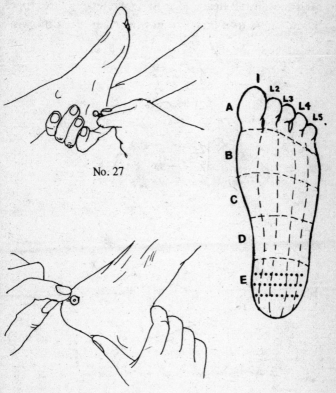

No. 27

No. 26

Next, work the inside and outside of the heel. Employ the main grip, or the instrument, see pictures No. 29 and No. 30. This area corresponds to the lower front and back, including the sex glands. Remember to work and to reach each spot in the area at least twice, preferably three times, but not more than that, except where indicated otherwise.

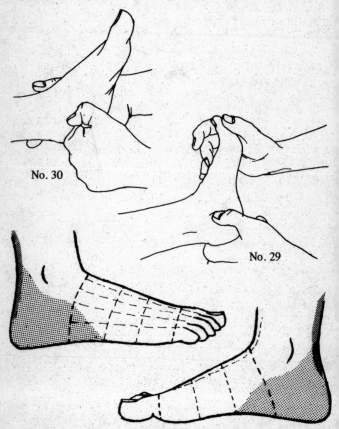

No. 30

No. 29

See the dotted line on top of the foot (at No. 36) where it joins the leg. Use the main grip or instrument, gently; see picture No. 28.

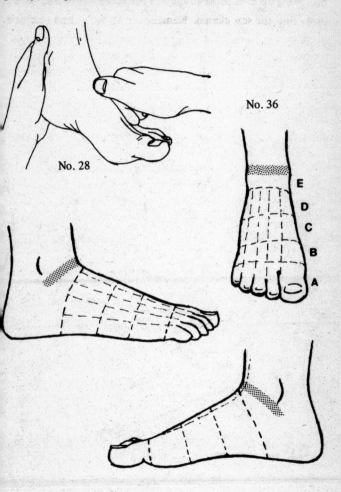

No. 36

No. 28

Next, check and stimulate the bony edge of the heel. Press hard with the main grip or instrument.

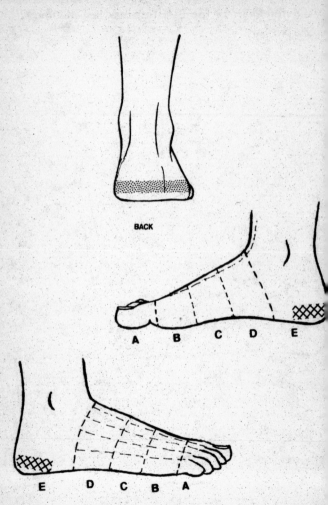

BACK

A  B  C  D  E

E  D  C  B  A

Now squeeze the Achilles' tendon (the cord in back of the heel) and the area next to it, strongly. Use thumb and forefinger or use 2 instruments, see picture No. 33 and No. 34.

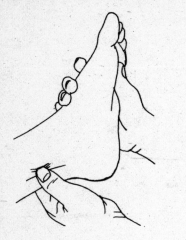

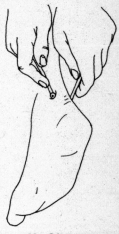

No. 33

No. 34

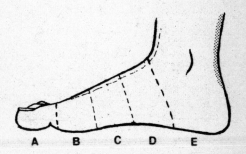

A    B    C    D    E

Last we employ the three relaxation grips. First twist your foot three times each way, see pictures No. 35, No. 36 and No. 37.

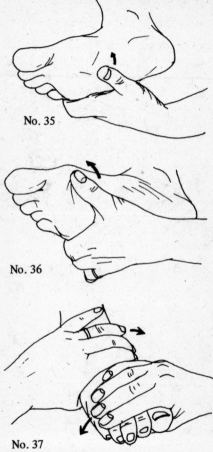

No. 35

No. 36

No. 37
Helping others

Then do the big toe circling until the toe feels loose. See picture No. 38.

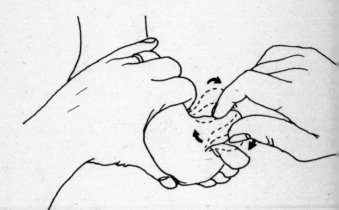

No. 38

Finally, rotate your foot from the ankle in a wide circle until it feels loose, see picture No. 39 and No. 40.

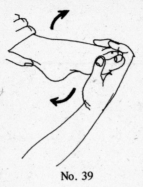

No. 39

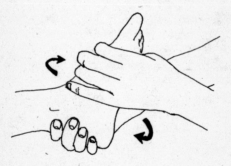

No. 40 Helping someone else

For the Wind Up inhale *deeply* six times, see picture No. 41. Always treat both feet. For tender points you have discovered, see the Condition Treatment Routine on page 77 and proceed accordingly.

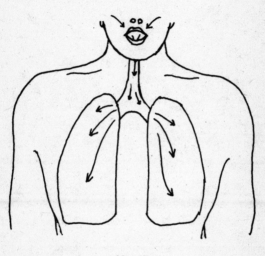

No. 41

# THE MAINTENANCE ROUTINE

Employ every second day. Once a week, replace it with the Check-Out Routine. Rub feet vigorously. Start at the X., see picture No. 52, main grip. Use the instrument for the thyroid detour and big toe, see pictures No. 11, No. 12 and No. 13.

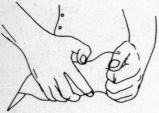

No. 11

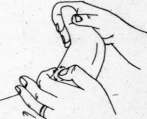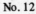

No. 12

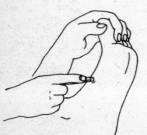

No. 13

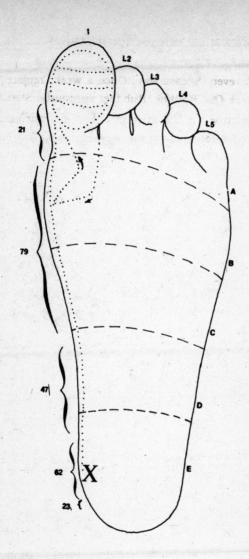

Now do the toe twist on the four small toes. Hold each toe firmly by the sides and twist, next hold top and bottom and twist. Do each toe in two sections. See picture No. 42.

No. 42

Employ either the knuckle of the thumb or the knuckles of the index and middle fingers, the double or single thumb or the instrument, see pictures No. 21, No. 22, No. 23, No. 24 and No. 25. Work from the ball of the foot to where the heel starts.

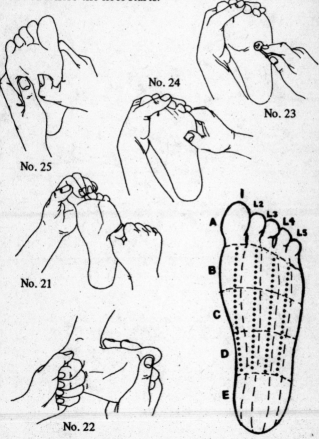

No. 24

No. 23

No. 25

No. 21

No. 22

Next, do the inside and outside of the heel. Employ either the side knuckle, the main grip, or the instrument, see pictures No. 29, No. 30 and No. 31. Then treat the Achilles' tendon, see picture No. 33.

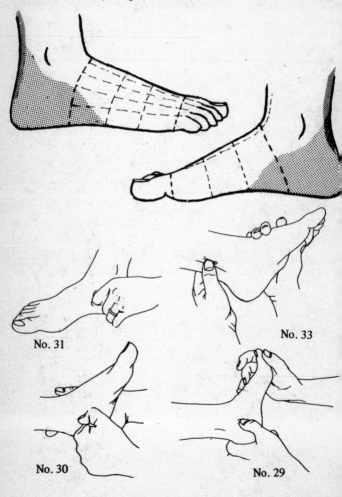

No. 31

No. 33

No. 30

No. 29

Last, employ the three relaxation grips. Twist the foot. See pictures No. 35, No. 36 and No. 37.

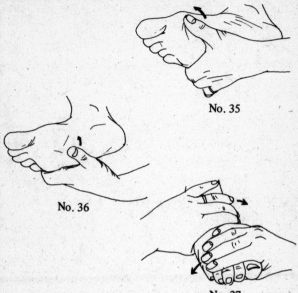

No. 35

No. 36

No. 37

Circle the big toe until it feels loose, see picture No. 38

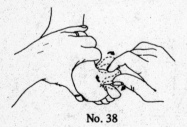

No. 38

Rotate the foot from the ankle in a wide circle until it feels loose, see pictures No. 39 and No. 40.

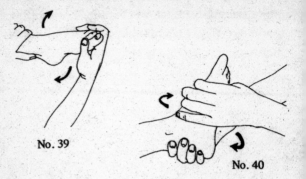

No. 39

No. 40

For the Wind Up inhale deeply 6 times, see picture No. 41. Always treat both feet.

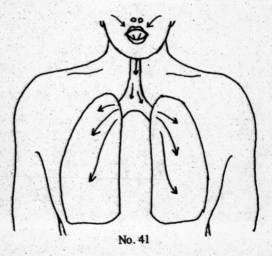

No. 41

## THE PICK-UP ROUTINE

Employ whenever you feel tired or worn out. Rub feet vigorously. Start on the underside of the big toe, the pituitary area. Employ the main grip, preferably with the instrument, see pictures No. 23 and No. 24. Proceed to the area corresponding to the thyroid gland. Next cover the adrenal and pancreas areas.

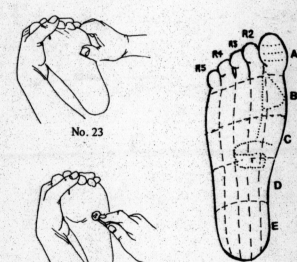

No. 23

No. 24

Next, work the inside and outside of the heel. Employ the side knuckle, the main grip, or the instrument, see pictures No. 29, No. 30 and No. 31. Then treat the Achilles' tendon, see picture No. 33

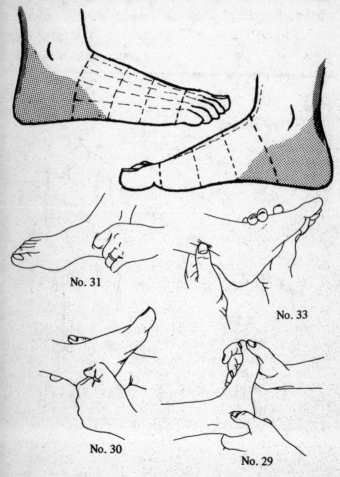

No. 31

No. 33

No. 30

No. 29

Last, employ the three relaxation grips. Twist the foot. See pictures No. 35, No. 36 and No. 37.

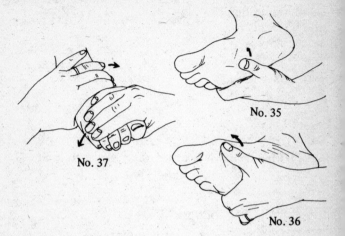

No. 35

No. 37

No. 36

Circle the big toe until it feels loose, see picture No. 38.

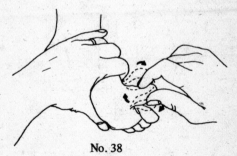

No. 38

Rotate the foot from the ankle.

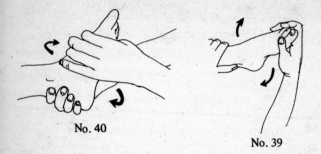

No. 40

No. 39

For the wind up inhale deeply 6 times. See picture No. 41.

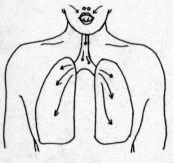

No. 41

Always treat both feet. Do not forget your weekly
Check-Out Routine.

# THE CONDITION TREATMENT ROUTINE

For upcoming or existing conditions. You have discovered one or several sore spots. Try to identify the source by the area where pain is located. See the big map. Check the corresponding pages and proceed accordingly. If you cannot identify the pain, just treat according to area instructions. If that does not help soon, see your doctor. Do not forget your weekly Check-Out Routine.

continued on page 83

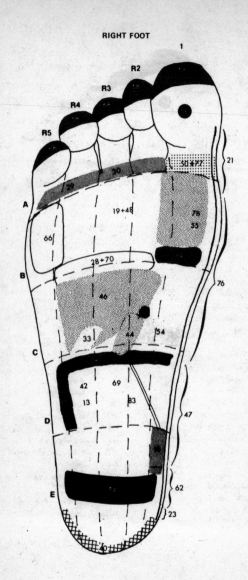

RIGHT FOOT

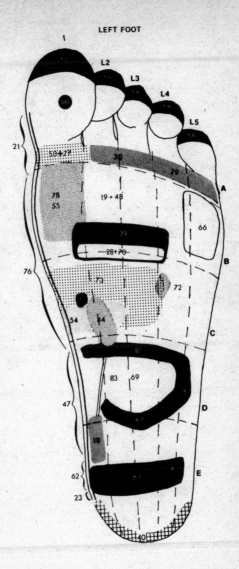

LEFT FOOT

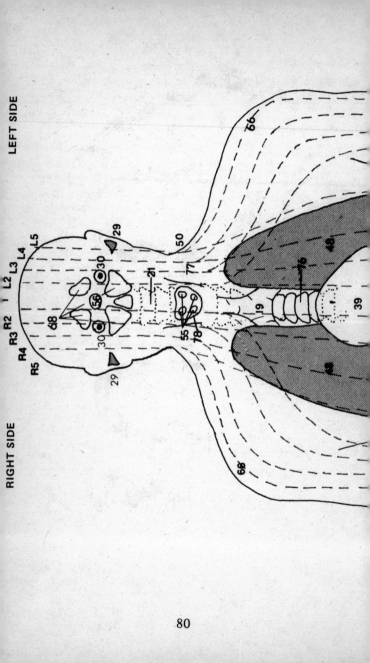

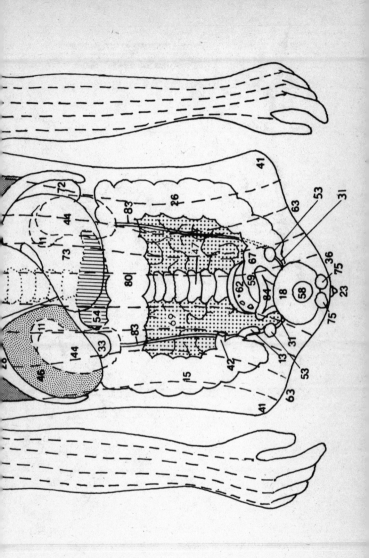

The press points for both the inside and
outside of the heels are the same on both
feet; always work on both feet.

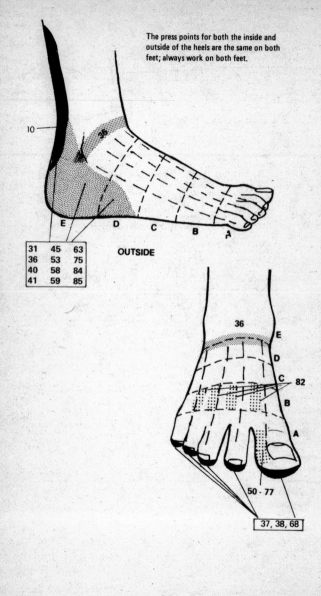

10

36

| E | D | C | B | A |

| 31 | 45 | 63 |
|----|----|----|
| 36 | 53 | 75 |
| 40 | 58 | 84 |
| 41 | 59 | 85 |

**OUTSIDE**

36

E
D
C — 82
B
A

50 - 77

37, 38, 68

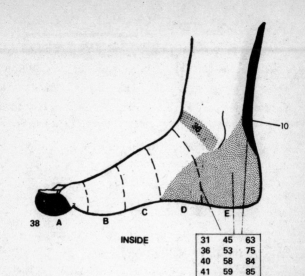

38 A    B    C    D    E

**INSIDE**

| 31 | 45 | 63 |
|----|----|----|
| 36 | 53 | 75 |
| 40 | 58 | 84 |
| 41 | 59 | 85 |

For numbers 10 to 49, see page 77.

| 30. | Neck |
| 31. | Nerve |
| 32. | Nervous Tension |
| 33. | Ovaries |
| 34. | Pancreas gland |
| 35. | Parathyroid glands |
| 36. | Pituitary gland |
| 37. | Press Points |
| 38. | Prostate gland |
| 39. | Rectum |
| 40. | Relaxation routine |
| 41. | Rheumatism |
| 42. | Sacrum |
| 43. | Sciatic nerve |
| 44. | Senility |
| 65. | Sex glands and organs |
| 66. | Shoulder |
| 67. | Sigmoid Colon |
| 68. | Sinus opening or cavity |
| 69. | Small intestines |
| 70. | Solar plexus |
| 71. | Spinal column |
| 72. | Spleen |
| 73. | Stomach |
| 74. | Teeth |
| 75. | Testes |
| 76. | Thoracic vertebrae |
| 77. | Throat |
| 78. | Thyroid gland |
| 79. | Tired? |
| 80. | Transverse colon |
| 81. | Ulcers |
| 82. | Upper torso |
| 83. | Ureter tubes |
| 84. | Uterus |
| 85. | Varicose veins |
| 86. | Weight control |

## THE MATURE PEOPLE ROUTINE

The purpose of this routine is to delay the signs and effects of aging. One day, you employ the Maintenance Routine. See page 66. The next day you use the Pick-Up Routine. See page 73. That is all you do: one day the Maintenance Routine, the next day the Pick-Up Routine. Once a week the Check-Out Routine should replace the Pick-Up Routine.

## THE RELAXATION ROUTINE

For nervous tension, mental and emotional stress. Employ the three Relaxation Routines at least three times daily, see pages 42, 43, 44, 45 and 46. Use these more often if necessary. Also, employ the Maintenance Routine, page 66 every second day for two weeks; after that, daily. Once a week the Check-Out Routine should replace the Maintenance Routine.

# PART IV

# HOW TO TREAT THE DIFFERENT AREAS
# OF THE BODY

10. Achilles' tendon: The thickest and strongest tendon, about 6 inches long, extending upward from the bac of the heel. It should be pliable.

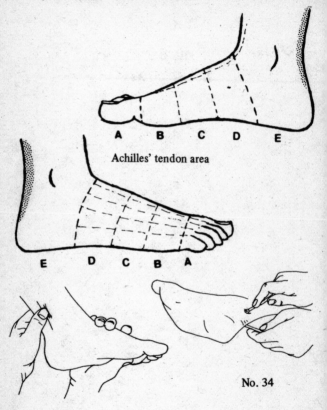

Achilles' tendon area

No. 33

No. 34

If your leg gets tired in the unaccustomed position, just switch feet as necessary.

11. **Adrenals:** Small glands located above each kidney. They are also called suprarenal glands. They are often helpful in controlling asthma.

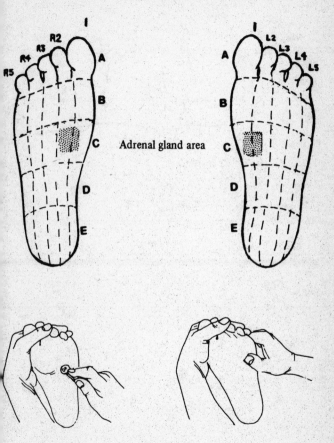

Adrenal gland area

No. 23 & No. 24

12. Anemia: A blood deficiency. Check spleen for tenderness.

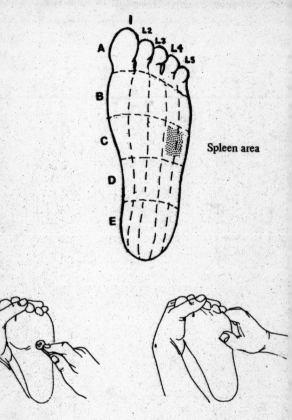

Spleen area

No. 23          No. 24

If your leg gets tired in the unaccustomed position, just switch feet as necessary.

13. **Appendix:** Lower right of the abdomen. When infected, may cause fever, pain, or nausea. See doctor at once. Treating press points will cause no harm.

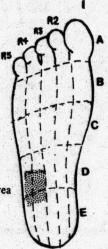

Appendix area. Same area as ileo-cecal valve

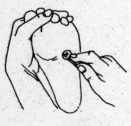

No. 23

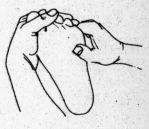

No. 24

14. Arthritis or rheumatic disease: There are over 60 varieties, from mild to crippling. Work each and every spot on both feet, taking special care of tender spots. For possible results you generally have to treat for quite a while. Follow beginner's Break-In Routine, page 18 then employ the Check-Out Routine daily. Page 47.

15. Ascending colon: See Colon No. 24, page 96.

16. Asthma: A respiratory disorder. It is often an allergy when bronchial. Work on the adrenal and other glands, include lungs. It could be helpful.

17. Backbone: See Spine No. 71, page 140.

If your leg gets tired in the unaccustomed position, just switch feet as necessary.

19. Bronchial tubes connect the trachea (windpipe) to the
    lungs. When necessary, treat entire area.

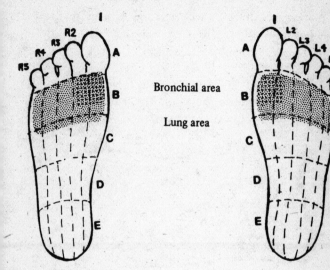

Bronchial area

Lung area

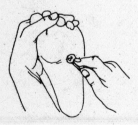

No. 23

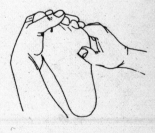

No. 24

18. **Bladder:** The expandable sac for the temporary retention of urine. Inflammation causes the repeated need to urinate. A few treatments will take care of it. If bleeding occurs, see doctor. Treat kidney and bladder areas in both feet. Check heel and Achilles' tendon for tender spots.

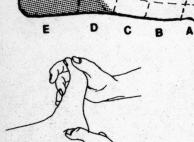

A    B    C    D    E

E    D    C    B    A

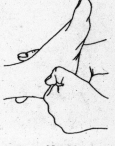

No. 29                              No. 30

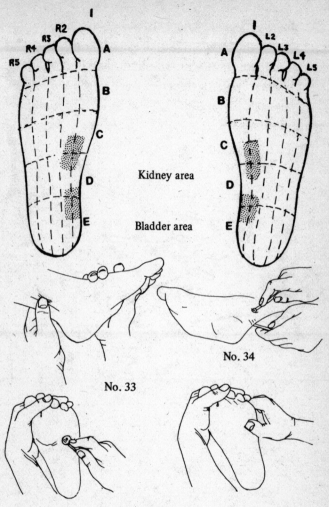

Kidney area

Bladder area

No. 33

No. 34

No. 23 & No. 24

20. Bursitis: Inflammation of the bursa. A pouch or sac containing a lubricating fluid located at certain points of friction, permits free motion. Painful when inflamed in shoulder, hip, knee, etc. Check glands and organs. Work on the corresponding press points for shoulder, hip, knee, etc.

Outside area both feet
Hip, Knee and leg area.

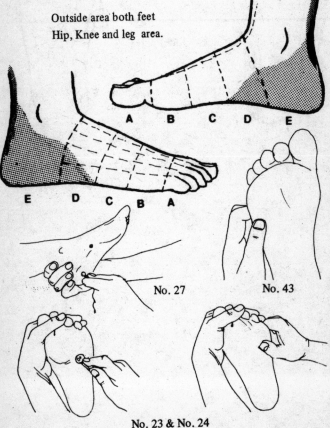

No. 27

No. 43

No. 23 & No. 24

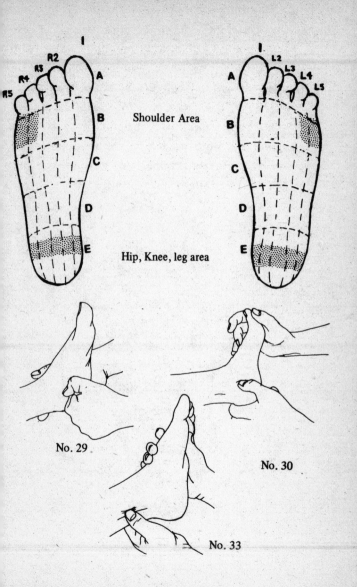

Shoulder Area

Hip, Knee, leg area

No. 29

No. 30

No. 33

24. Colon: The storage and dehydrating organ. The "ascending" colon (see No. 15 below) starts on the right side of the body; as it crosses over to the left side, it is called "transverse" colon (see No. 80 below), then "descending" colon (see No. 26 below) and finally "sigmoid" colon (see No. 67 below). Give this area a good workout when needed, paying special attention to sore spots. Remember, they are warning signals and should disappear after a few treatments.

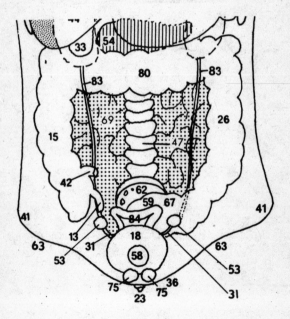

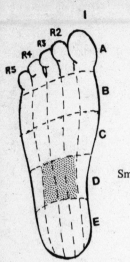
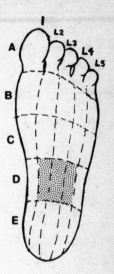

R1
R2
R3
R4
R5
A
B
C
D
E

I
L2
L3
L4
L5
A
B
C
D
E

Small intestine area

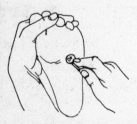
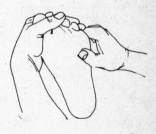

No. 23 & No. 24

21. Cervical vertebrae: Neck segment of spine. See spine No. 71, page 140.

22. Circulatory system: Work both feet thoroughly. Better circulation improves health. Follow beginner's Break-In Routine, page 18.

23. Coccyx: Tail bone, see Spine No. 71, page 140.

25. Constipation: Infrequent or difficult bowel movement. There are many possible reasons. When you employ your weekly Check-Out Routine, pay special attention to tender spots corresponding to the intestines, colon, liver, rectum, and related areas.

26. Descending colon: See Colon No. 24, page 96.

If your leg gets tired in the unaccustomed position, just switch feet as necessary.

27. Diabetes: Malfunctioning of the pancreas gland. Treatment produces results more often in adults. Check for possible change in quantity of insulin needed.

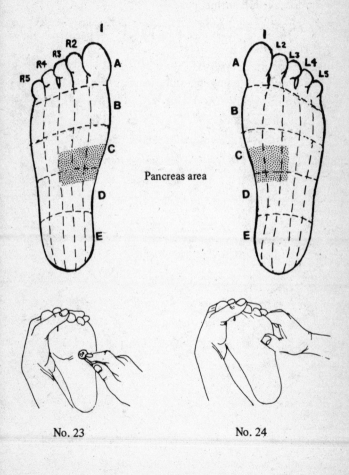

Pancreas area

No. 23

No. 24

28. Diaphragm: Chief breathing muscle which separates chest from abdomen.

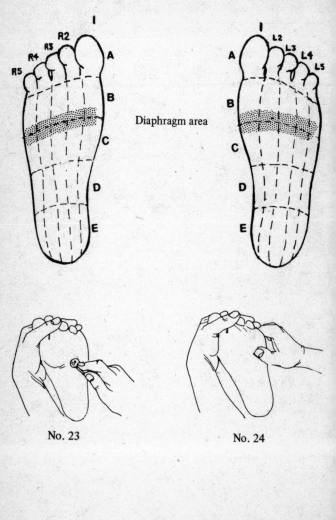

Diaphragm area

No. 23          No. 24

31. Fallopian Tubes: Also known as oviducts, passage-
    ways of egg cells to the uterus.

32. Fatigue: See tired No. 79, page 147.

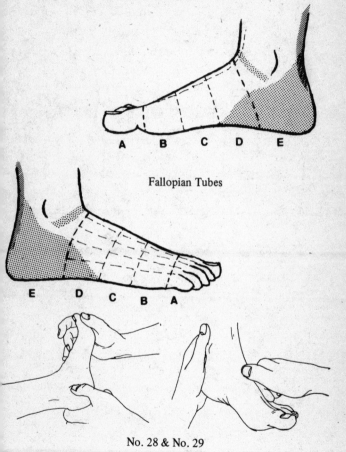

Fallopian Tubes

No. 28 & No. 29

29. Ear: For most problems work between third and fourth, and fourth and fifth toes. Use finger, thumb, or preferably an instrument, to get into every nook and cranny. Then use the three-finger grip on "ledge" at base of toes, and move around. You are bound to find the tender press points that have to be worked out. To obtain improvement, always work both feet.

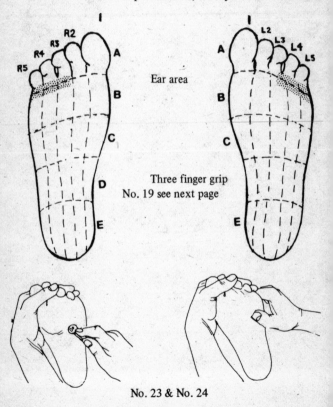

Ear area

Three finger grip
No. 19 see next page

No. 23 & No. 24

30. Eyes are helped often by a treatment quite similar to the one employed for the ears. Basic press points are located between the second and third toes. Follow instructions given for ears, see previous page.

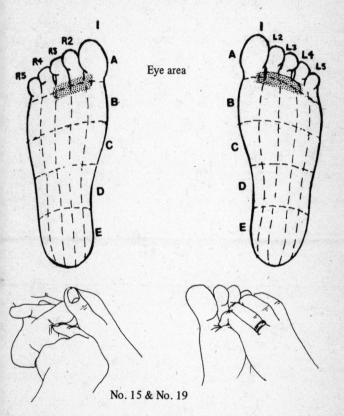

Eye area

No. 15 & No. 19

If your leg gets tired in the unaccustomed position, just switch feet as necessary.

33. Gall bladder: A small pouch-like organ, beneath right lobe of liver, which stores bile.

34. Gall Stones: Treating liver and gall bladder area often proves successful.

35. Glands: Find under A for Adrenal, T for Thyroid, etc.

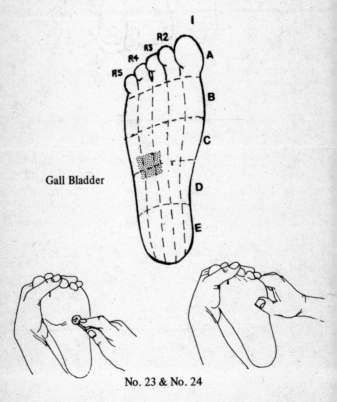

Gall Bladder

No. 23 & No. 24

## 36. Groin: Lowest part of torso where it joins the legs.

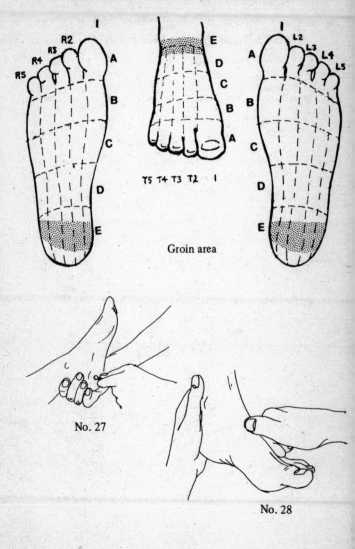

Groin area

No. 27

No. 28

105

37. Hayfever: Annually recurring allergic reaction which affects membranes of the eyes and nasal passages. Work faithfully and often on the designated areas and tender spots, and you will find relief.

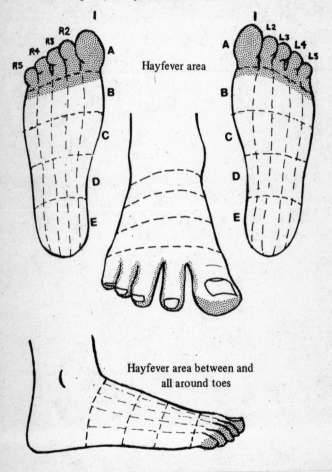

Hayfever area

Hayfever area between and all around toes

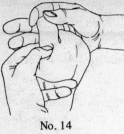

No. 14

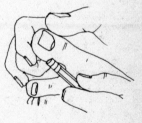

No. 17

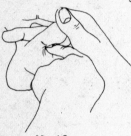

No. 15

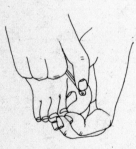

No. 18

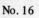

No. 16

38. Headaches: Differ in intensity and location. Start by looking for tender points in the big toes, tops and sides. Points where these connect with the foot and between other toes is also important. Make sure you reach all nooks and crannies. Do not give up after you find one spot. There are probably more than one demanding a good workout. Treat whenever necessary. Rotate your big toes in circles to the right and to the left. This relaxes the head. You will feel it. Next, start searching in other areas which could conceivably cause that headache, such as the stomach, colon, liver, etc. Best employ the Check-Out Routine.

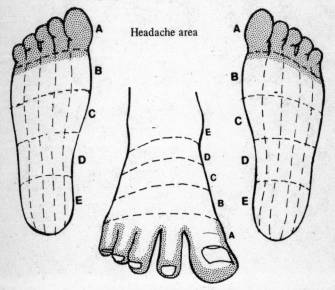

Headache area

Headache areas between and
all around toes, specially big toes

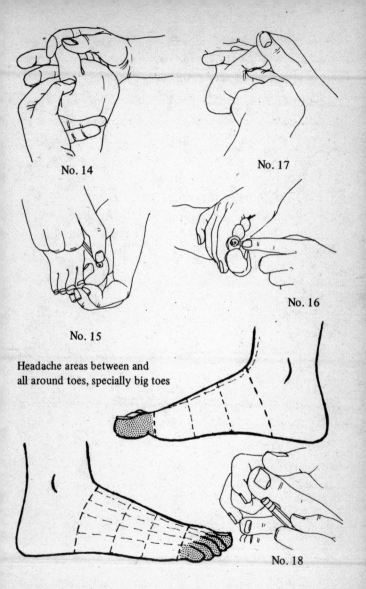

No. 14

No. 17

No. 15

No. 16

Headache areas between and
all around toes, specially big toes

No. 18

39. **Heart:** The muscular pump that keeps us going. Since it is located deep in the body, you really have to press hard to feel the tender spots.

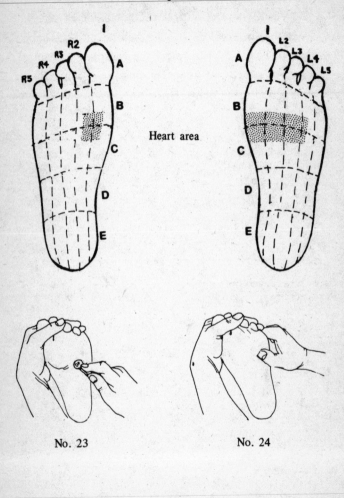

Heart area

No. 23

No. 24

41. Hips: See Bursitis No. 20, page 94 and see Sciatic nerve No. 63, page 130.

42. Ileo cecal valve: Controls the admission of semi-liquids into the colon. It is located next to the appendix on the right side below the waist line. If painful, see your doctor at once. Treating press points cannot harm and often helps. Grips No. 23 and No. 24 same as on page 110.

43. Intestines: See Colon No. 24 page 96 and Small Intestines No. 69, page 138.

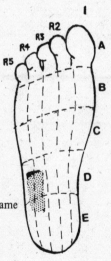

Ileo-cecal valve area same area as appendix

40. Hemorrhoids (Piles): Varicose veins in and around the rectal opening. If bleeding profusely, see your doctor.

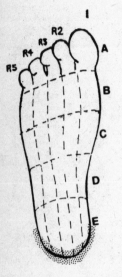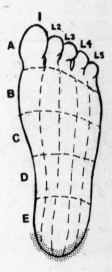

Hemorrhoidal area, the
outer edge of the heel.

If your leg gets tired in the unaccustomed position, just switch feet as necessary.

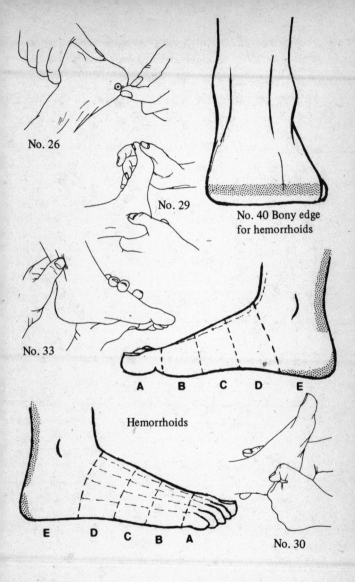

No. 26

No. 29

No. 40 Bony edge
for hemorrhoids

No. 33

A    B    C    D    E

Hemorrhoids

E    D    C    B    A

No. 30

44. **Kidneys:** A pair of bean-shaped glandular organs on both sides of the body at the back of the abdominal cavity. They filter out impurities. They are subject to kidney stones, infection, inflammation, etc. Treat tender points gently during break-in time.

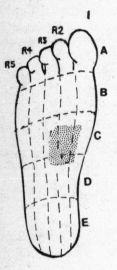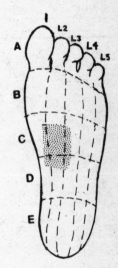

Kidney area

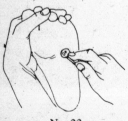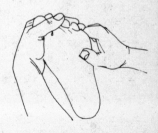

No. 23            No. 24

46. Liver: Largest glandular organ which is essentially on right side. Chemically, it is the most versatile organ. Always check for tenderness. Treat gently during break-in time.

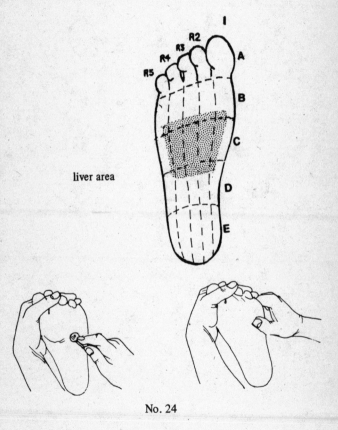

liver area

No. 24

45. Knee and Leg: See Bursitis No. 20 page 94.

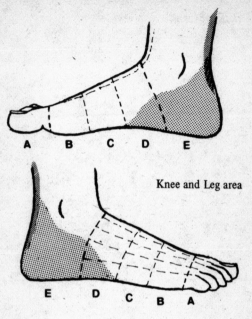

Knee and Leg area

No. 45

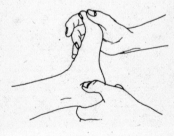

No. 29

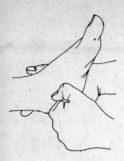

No. 30

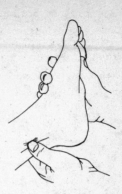

No. 33

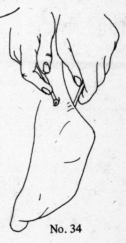

No. 31

No. 34

47. Lumbar vertebrae: See Spine, No. 71, page 140. Lumbar region which is from slightly above to slightly below waist line. When treating, always check related areas, including Kidneys.

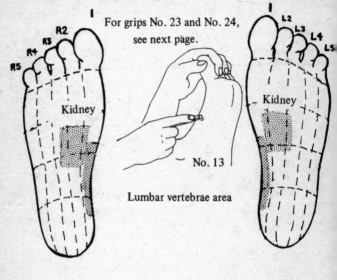

For grips No. 23 and No. 24,
see next page.

Kidney

Kidney

No. 13

Lumbar vertebrae area

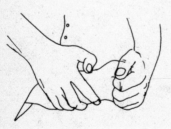

No. 11

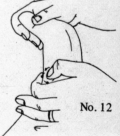

No. 12

48. Lungs: Organs of respiration on either side of chest cavity.

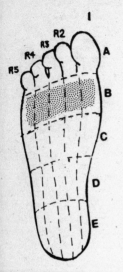
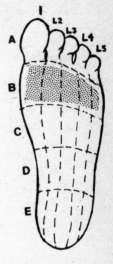

Lung area

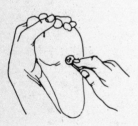
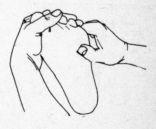

No. 23 & No. 24

49. Mental health: Nervous tension: See No. 52, this page.

51. Nerve: Cordlike fiber composed of microscopic filaments, serving as the path of nerve impulses.

52. Nervous Tension: Mental and emotional stress. Employ Relaxation Routine, page 84.

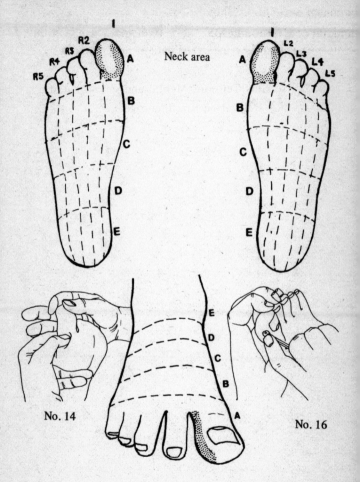

Neck area

R1
R2
R3
R4
R5
A
B
C
D
E

L2
L3
L4
L5
A
B
C
D
E
I

No. 14

No. 16

E
D
C
B
A

Neck area

53. **Ovaries:** Female glands which provide egg cells and secrete hormones. Check their press point areas on both feet as well as the thyroid gland areas on both feet.

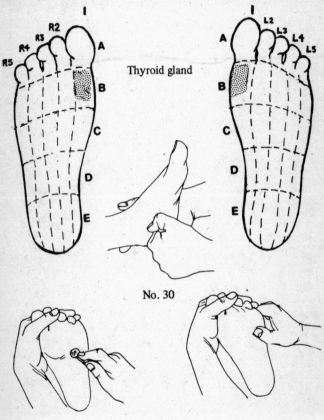

Thyroid gland

No. 30

No. 23 & No. 24

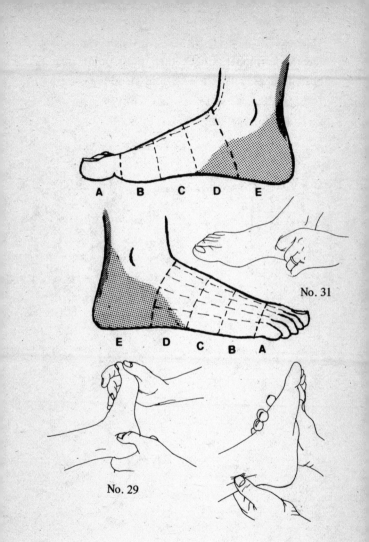

A   B   C   D   E

E   D   C   B   A

No. 31

No. 29

No. 33

123

54. Pancreas gland: Secretes insulin and digestive enzymes. Work tender spots in the area. Several different organs are overlapping here, so it is difficult to know which is responsible for the tenderness. Just work it out. In case of diabetes, check No. 27, page 99.

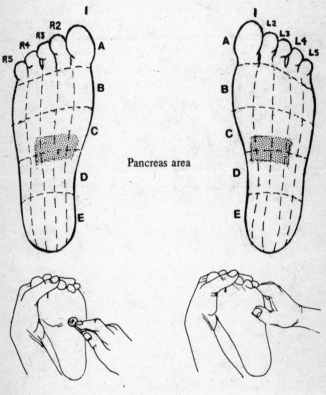

Pancreas area

No. 23 & No. 24

55. Parathyroid glands: All four are supposed to be imbedded in the thyroid gland. Sometimes one or more are misplaced. Responsible for the calcium in the blood. They benefit from treating the thyroid gland, but may need a little firmer pressure.

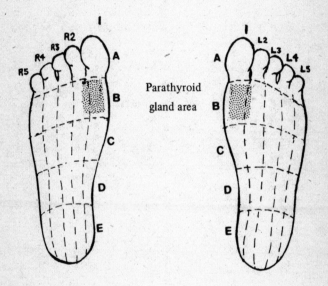

Parathyroid gland area

Grips No. 23 and No. 24 see previous page.

If your leg gets tired in the unaccustomed position, just switch feet as necessary.

56. Pituitary gland: Known as the "master gland" and located at the base of the brain. The press point is located close to the center underneath each big toe. If you cannot press hard enough with your thumb to feel it, use an instrument. You should *always* feel your pituitary gland while pressing.

57. Press points: Are located in the hands, as well as in the feet.

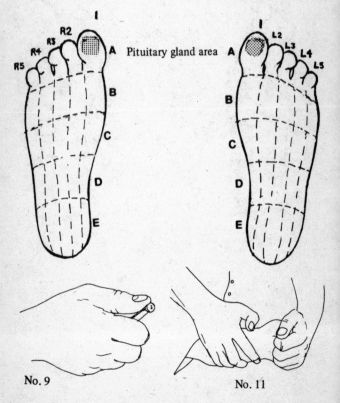

Pituitary gland area

No. 9          No. 11

60. Relaxation Routine: See page 84.

61. Rheumatism: See Arthritis No. 14 page 90.

62. Sacrum: Curved bone just above tailbone (coccyx).
    See Spine, No. 71, page 140.

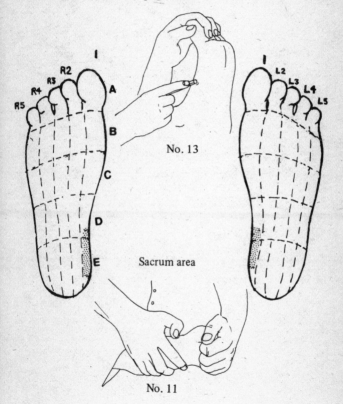

No. 13

Sacrum area

No. 11

58. Prostate gland: Largest male sex gland located in front of rectum. Press point treatments for complications generally prove successful.

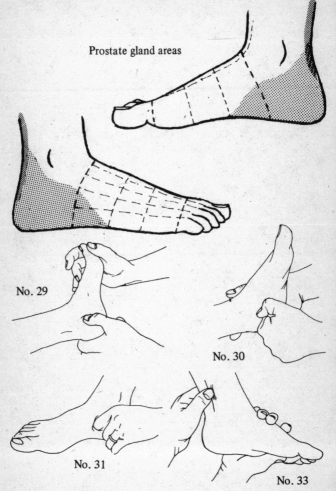

Prostate gland areas

No. 29

No. 30

No. 31

No. 33

## 59. Rectum: End of large intestine.

The grips are the same for page 128 and page 129.

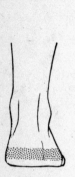

BACK

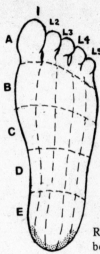

Rectum area and
bony edge

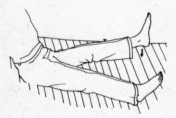

No. 32

If your leg gets tired in the unaccustomed position, just switch feet
as necessary.

63. Sciatic (hip joint) Nerve: Is the largest nerve cord in the body. When inflamed, it is painful, but generally responds well to Press Point Therapy.

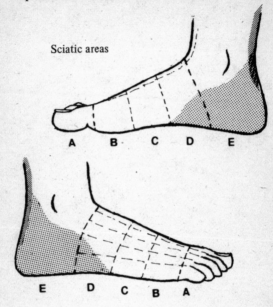

Sciatic areas

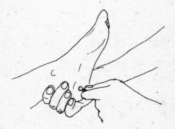

No. 27

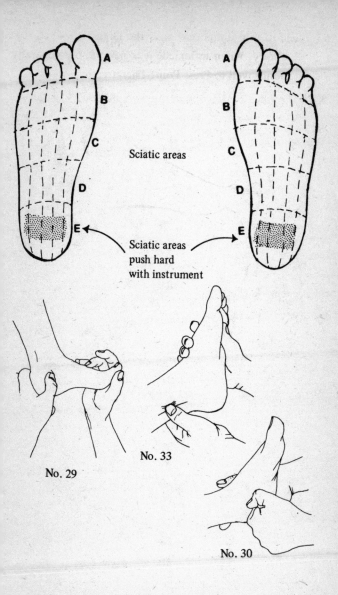

Sciatic areas

Sciatic areas
push hard
with instrument

No. 29

No. 33

No. 30

131

64. Senility: Mental and physical infirmity, due to advanced age. See the Mature People Routine, page 84.

65. Sex glands and organs: In the female — fallopian tubes, ovaries and uterus. In the male — prostate gland, testicles and seminal vesicles.

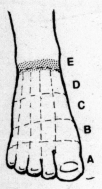

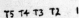
T5  T4  T3  T2  1

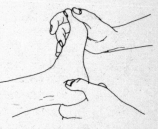
No. 28

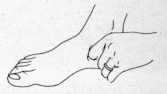
No. 29

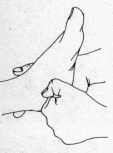
No. 30

No. 31

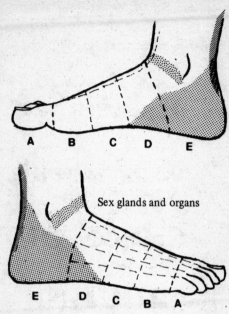

Sex glands and organs

A B C D E

E D C B A

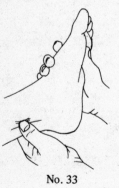

No. 33

# Remember

## your weekly

# CHECK-OUT

# ROUTINE

66. Shoulder: See Bursitis No. 20, page 94.

67. Sigmoid Colon: See Colon No. 24, page 96.

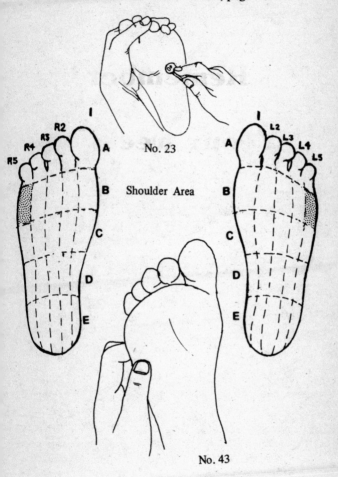

No. 23

Shoulder Area

No. 43

68. Sinus opening or cavity: Four pairs of paranasal sinuses concern us. These membrane-lined cavities around the nose are subject to inflammation, or head cold, called sinusitis. Work faithfully and often on the designated areas and tender spots, and you will find relief.

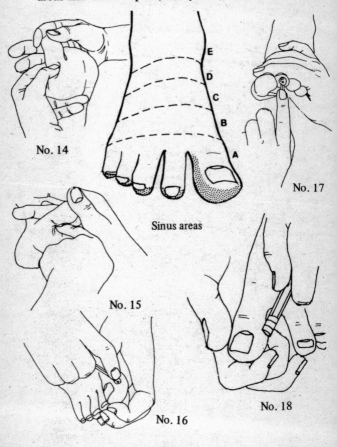

No. 14

No. 17

No. 15

No. 16

No. 18

Sinus areas

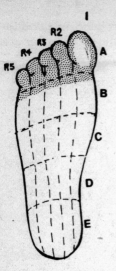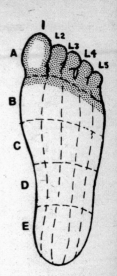

Sinus areas both feet

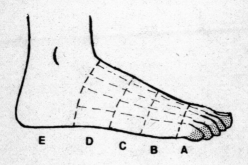

69. Small intestines: Where digestion is completed and most nutrients are absorbed.

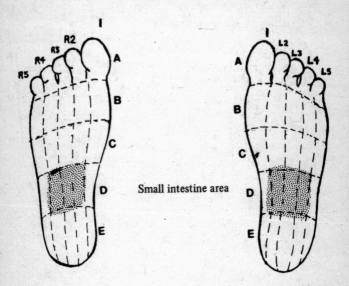

Small intestine area

For grips No. 23 and No. 24, see next page

If your leg gets tired in the unaccustomed position, just switch feet as necessary.

70. Solar plexus (pit of stomach): Network for the sympathetic nervous system, located behind the stomach and in front of the diaphragm.

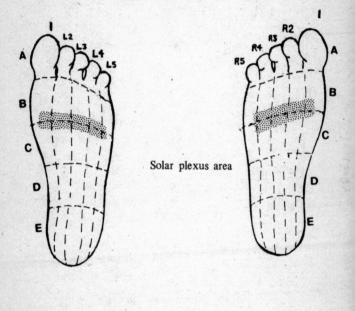

Solar plexus area

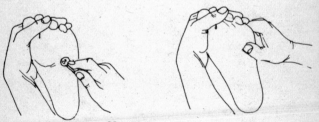

No. 23 & No. 24

71. Spinal column, or backbone: Cervical vertebrae, thoracic vertebrae, lumbar vertebrae, sacrum and coccyx (tail bone).

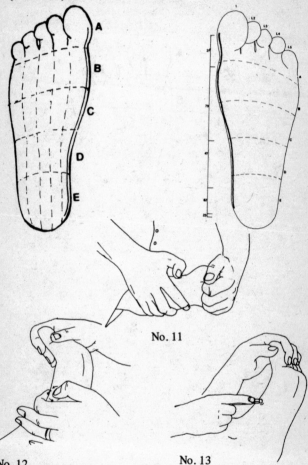

No. 11

No. 12

No. 13

72. Spleen: Takes in the dead red cells. When area is tender it could either be an anemic condition or malfunctioning of some other nearby organ or gland.

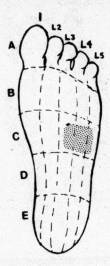

Spleen area

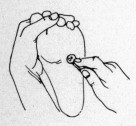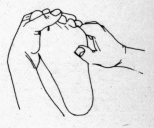

No. 23 & No. 24

73. Stomach: Biggest bulge in the digestive tract. It is located behind the ribs — not under or below the navel. Ulcers develop for many reasons. Depending on its condition, treatment may be painful. Brace yourself and work it out, as it is well worth it.

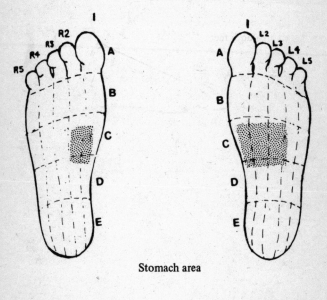

Stomach area

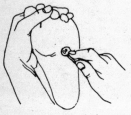 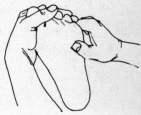

No. 23 & No. 24

74. Teeth: Have regular checkups — an infected tooth may cause a painful reaction anywhere in the body.

75. Testes: Testicles — primary male sex glands.

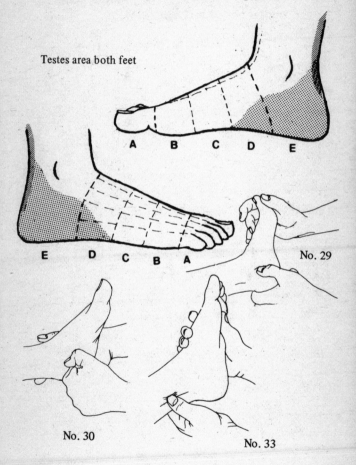

Testes area both feet

A   B   C   D   E

E   D   C   B   A

No. 29

No. 30

No. 33

76. Thoracic vertebrae: See Spine No. 71 page 140.

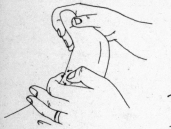

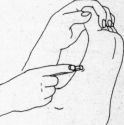

No. 12          No. 13

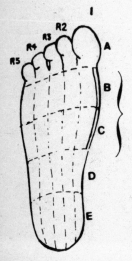

Thoracic vertebrae

77. Throat: In back of the mouth. It is also called the Pharynx.

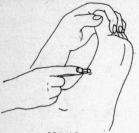

No. 13

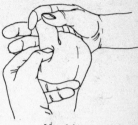

No. 14

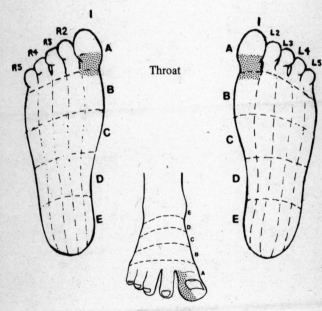

Throat

Throat area

78. Thyroid gland: Located in neck and covers the front and sides of windpipe (trachea). It is related to iodine supply and metabolism.

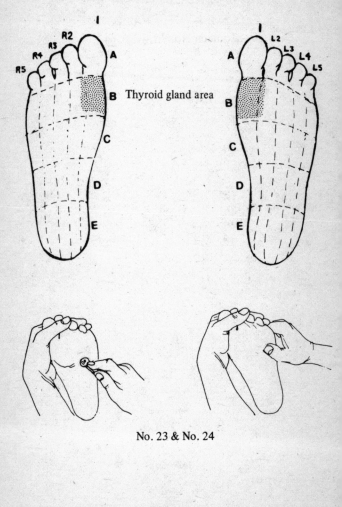

Thyroid gland area

No. 23 & No. 24

79. Tired? Do the Pick-Up Routine which revitalizes, see page 73.

80. Transverse colon: See Colon No. 24, page 96.

81. Ulcers: See Stomach No. 73, page 142.

## 82. Upper torso

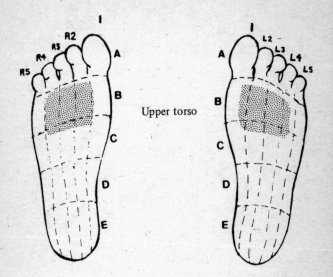

Upper torso

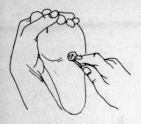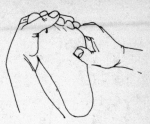

No. 23 & No. 24

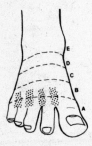

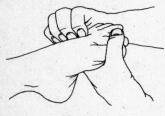

No. 20

83. Ureter tubes: The urine passes through these from the kidneys to the bladder.

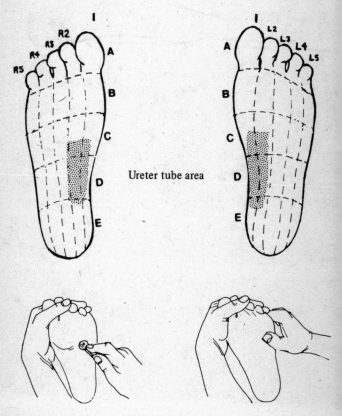

Ureter tube area

No. 23 & No. 24

## 84. Uterus: The Womb.

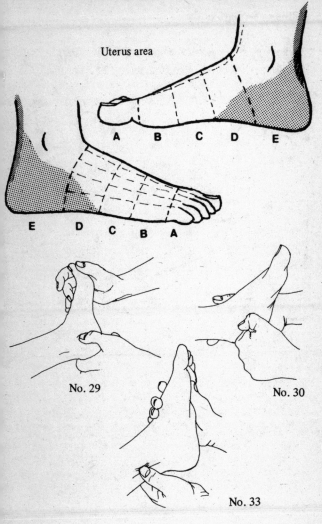

Uterus area

A B C D E

E D C B A

No. 29

No. 30

No. 33

85. Varicose veins: Swollen, dilated and contorted veins mostly in the legs.

86. Weight control: Stimulating the various glands helps. Employ the Pick-Up Routine, page 73 and eat sensibly.

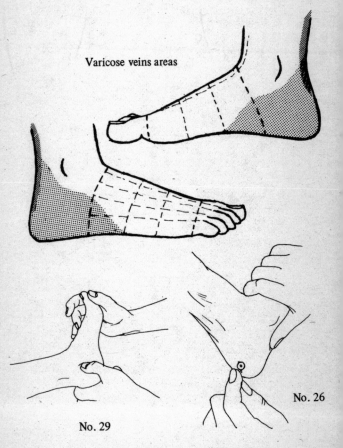

Varicose veins areas

No. 29

No. 26

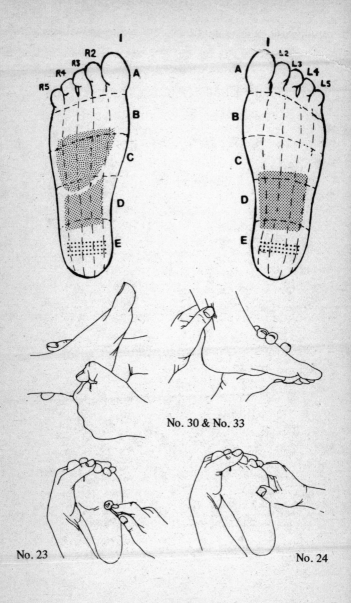

No. 30 & No. 33

No. 23

No. 24

153

# INDEX

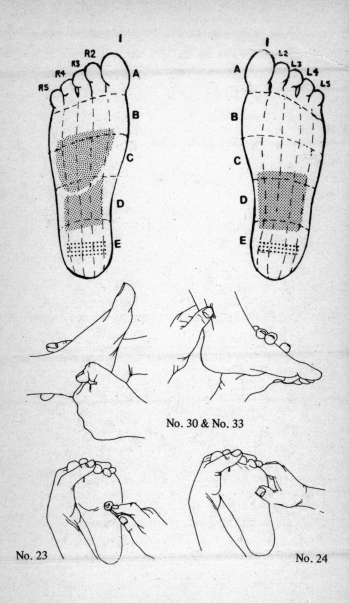

No. 30 & No. 33

No. 23

No. 24

153

# INDEX

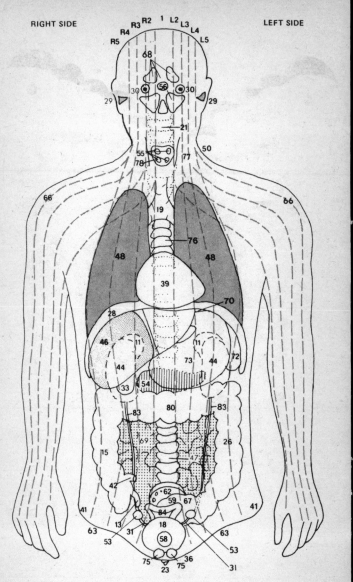

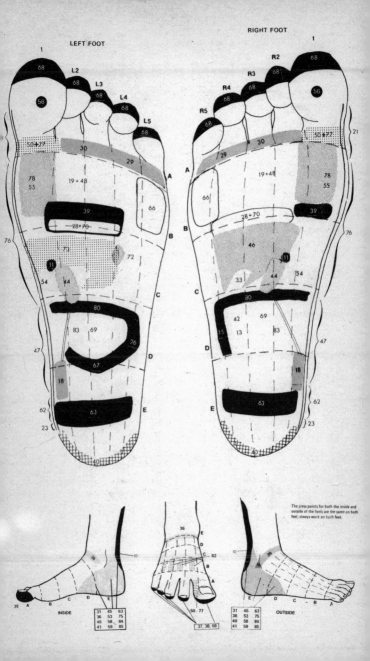

| | | | |
|---|---|---|---|
| 10. | Achilles tendon | 49. | Mental health, nerve tension |
| 11. | Adrenals | 50. | Neck |
| 12. | Anemia | 51. | Nerve |
| 13. | Appendix | 52. | Nervous Tension |
| 14. | Arthritis | 53. | Ovaries |
| 15. | Ascending colon | 54. | Pancreas gland |
| 16. | Asthma | 55. | Parathyroid glands |
| 17. | Backbone, see spine | 56. | Pituitary gland |
| 18. | Bladder | 57. | Press Points |
| 19. | Bronchial tubes | 58. | Prostate gland |
| 20. | Bursitis | 59. | Rectum |
| 21. | Cervical vertebrae | 60. | Relaxation routine |
| 22. | Circulatory system | 61. | Rheumatism |
| 23. | Coccyx | 62. | Sacrum |
| 24. | Colon | 63. | Sciatic nerve |
| 25. | Constipation | 64. | Senility |
| 26. | Descending colon | 65. | Sex glands and organs |
| 27. | Diabetes | 66. | Shoulder |
| 28. | Diaphragm | 67. | Sigmoid Colon |
| 29. | Ear | 68. | Sinus opening or cavity |
| 30. | Eyes | 69. | Small intestines |
| 31. | Fallopian tubes | 70. | Solar plexus |
| 32. | Fatigue | 71. | Spinal column |
| 33. | Gall bladder | 72. | Spleen |
| 34. | Gall Stones | 73. | Stomach |
| 35. | Glands | 74. | Teeth |
| 36. | Groin | 75. | Testes |
| 37. | Hayfever | 76. | Thoracic vertebrae |
| 38. | Headaches | 77. | Throat |
| 39. | Heart | 78. | Thyroid gland |
| 40. | Hemorrhoids (Piles) | 79. | Tired? |
| 41. | Hips | 80. | Transverse colon |
| 42. | Ileo cecal valve | 81. | Ulcers |
| 43. | Intestines, see small | 82. | Upper torso |
| 44. | Kidneys | 83. | Ureter tubes |
| 45. | Knee and Leg | 84. | Uterus |
| 46. | Liver | 85. | Varicose veins |
| 47. | Lumbar vertebrae (Lumbago) | 86. | Weight control |
| 48. | Lungs | | |